I0135866

Alkaline Diet

Simple And Tasty Recipes With A Meal Plan To Reduce
Inflammation And Improve Your Health

*(Green Smoothies Made From Alkaline Plants For Optimal
Health)*

Marcus Bristow

TABLE OF CONTENT

Lifestyle Advice

Your lifestyle plays a significant role in your health status, especially with regard to the rH homeostasis within your body. There are numerous lifestyle habits and challenges that can lead to high levels of acidity in the body; therefore, it is crucial that we develop new healthy lifestyle habits to promote alkalinity, in addition to eating the correct foods. In this section, I will share seven life hacks that will assist in regulating your body's pH level.

Breathe

Do you know how to rrorerlu breathe? We've all been doing it since the day we were born, but many of us have developed poor habits and only get a small portion of the oxygen we need to

3

feed our hearts and brains, ensure that our metabolic processes function efficiently, and maintain a healthy alkaline body. Rapid, labored respiration is one of the most alkalinizing rashes available. Best of all, it is completely free and will also make you feel happier and harder.

Therefore, learn to breathe deeply by performing the mrle exercise:

Inhale for two counts, filling the lower rart of your lung frt, then the middle rart, and finally the upper rart.

Hold your breath for eight seconds. It may be difficult at the moment, but it will get easier.

Exhale slowly for four counts, emphasizing first the upper region of your lungs, then the middle, and finally the lower.

Then, repeat the process ten times.

Manage stress

In the modern era, the majority of us are subject to some degree of stress every single day of our lives; there is no way to avoid it. A certain amount of stress is actually healthy because it helps us feel both challenged and motivated. However, when stress levels become chronic, they place the body under incredible amounts of strain and cause a severe acid/alkaline imbalance as well as many other health issues.

Your digestive system shuts down in response to stress, limiting your body's ability to assimilate nutrients and leaving you more susceptible than ever to ill health. In addition, tre also interferes with our hormones, elevating levels of the tre hormone sortol and free radicals, which can cause cell damage, dementia, heart disease, and even cancer.

As you can imagine, it is crucial that you manage your stress level and learn effective stress-management techniques so that you can live your regular life without negative consequences. First, determine if there is a way for you to reduce your level of tension. This may entail delegating important tasks to those around you, taking time for yourself, or even occasionally saying "no."

Then determine which stress-management techniques accommodate your lifestyle the most. Take your time to find one that works for you, as there are many available. Mu reronal favorte include uoga, meditation, and ta chi, and when I find solace in my uoga practice, I am best able to relax and recharge. What would be your preferred activity?

Sleep

According to what I've heard, Elle MasPheron's favored aspect of the alkaline lifestyle is allowing herself the extra leeway she desires, and I couldn't agree with her more. Sleer is the body's way of repairing damaged tissues, recuperating, growing, and rebalancing the endocrinological system and rH balance. - If you're not getting enough sleep, you're not doing yourself any favors and keeping your body in an unhealthy state.

So, make reading your top priority! Write it in your calendar as you would any other important appointment, and adhere to it. You have a duty to yourself.

I expect to get approximately eight hours of sleep tonight. Your optimal quantity will vary depending on your individual requirements.

Chapter 1: Trigger Warning: The Origin Of Our Weight

Throughout your infancy or adolescence, you may have experienced periods of low self-confidence and lack of motivation. Or you could be an adult, self-sufficient male who once had everything under control but now struggles with sobriety and wishes to lose unhealthy weight.

Your journey up to this point has not been a waste of your life, as you may believe, but it has contributed significantly to the person who is in charge of not giving up! May I say, you can rest now? You can hold onto objects even when you are not physically grasping them. And this is likely why your weight is clinging to things you cannot see and are oblivious of, but have also not subconsciously let go of.

There are a variety of causes for holding onto memories, trauma, loss, shocks, rejection, and sadness, but your entire existence and its experiences may have shaped your relationship with food. And that is not at all terrible news. The good news is that it is possible to restore relationships in this life and in this world. We are granted a second chance, a third opportunity, and sometimes even a fourth chance.

On the contrary, you could be a person without such experience who simply acquired the weight. There is a strong possibility that your weight is not a problem, but you now view it as one and wish to lose weight. You still have the opportunity to better understand yourself and live a healthy existence.

The Weight Load Cannot Destroy You!

Your body will only dance to healthier rhythms if you pay attention to the musical notes it sends you. Our body gives us these "okay" and "not okay" signals. There are certain foods that you will embrace without question. However, you may develop an allergy to other substances. Similarly, you may experience some anxiety before beginning a particular diet. The notion of drinking juice three times a day may make you gag and curl your toes, but for the sake of "looking good," you are willing to endure something that makes you queasy.

Ask yourself the query, "Is this even worthwhile?" at every turn.

Remember that the burden that can overwhelm you is not your weight, but rather the burden of expectations, the burden of insecurities, and the burden of comparison.

The accomplishment of fitting into a bathing suit after an arduous process of rigorous exercise and fasting! Except when the sole purpose of this voyage was to fit into a bathing suit. Your motivation for dieting should precede your desire to diet. And as crucial as it is to look good, it is also essential to feel good. The pleasure derived from the thought of looking attractive is not eternal.

To be fit and healthy enough to run freely on the shore and play in the sand and waves, you must diet. Looking good to feel good is not completely irrelevant to this procedure. However, this limited perspective will only trap you in limitations.

What embarrasses you is probably not the number you see each morning on the scale. It is the gaze of persons you don't even know that pierces you. But have you ever considered that you allow it to penetrate you? Consider the inner child you are being harsh with when you are being cruel with yourself. But now you have the chance to get closer to yourself and make this process of being healthy successful.

Do not make isolation and anxiety your refuge. It is not your responsibility to battle the afflictions of others. Your only duty is to combat your own insecurities. Some days will be exceedingly challenging, while other days you will not even consider it.

A journey on the alkaline diet may not be right for you, and I am not here to force you to go on a diet. This book's sole purpose was to provide you with a balanced look at the pros and cons of everything you may encounter on this or any other diet.

Diet or no diet, we scramble to validate our emotions and view an improved version of ourselves from a distance. To get any closer to that version, we must exert great effort. But effort alone does not guarantee success.

The right quantity of work in the right direction, with the right knowledge, entails taking a break, rewinding so as not to discard everything we have learned, and creating something new by combining the modern and the ancient in order to survive in the present.

Being healthy is first and foremost a contest of the mind. Attempting to survive in a body that you do not want or like is a situation that dulls the intellect.

But surviving the affair of loving the same body and overcoming all odds is a feeling, a decision, an endeavor toward persuasion, and also a judgment at the same time.

Before commencing any diet, cancer patients should consult their physician or a dietitian about their nutritional needs.

People who are taking medications to treat osteoporosis, arthritis, urinary tract infections, kidney stones, headaches, or other conditions that are purportedly cured by alkaline diets should not stop taking their medications if they decide to attempt an alkaline diet.

Many protein and calcium sources that are allowed in moderation in other diets, such as lean meat or powdered milk, are not permitted in alkaline diet programs. Consequently, people who follow an alkaline diet must be careful to consume enough protein and calcium from the foods they do consume.

Alkaline diets are difficult for many people to adhere to, not only because of the restricted food options, but also because they make dining out and living with family members who do not follow the diet more difficult. In addition, since manufactured foods are prohibited, alkaline diets typically require more time and effort for meal preparation.

RISKS FACTOR

Long-term consumption of an alkaline diet can result in nutritional deficiencies due to a lack of calcium, protein, and essential fatty acids. In addition, individuals who discontinue the use of medications prescribed to treat conditions such as arthritis, cancer, diabetes, osteoporosis, or kidney stones because they believe an alkaline diet will suffice run the risk of experiencing a worsening of their symptoms. Dieters who purchase alkaline water or other alkaline supplements to supplement their diet risk being deceived by manufacturers who misbrand their products or make unsubstantiated health claims. In addition, the FDA reports that samples of so-called alkaline water have been found to contain salmonella and other pathogens.

WHAT TO EAT AND WHAT TO AVOID

What to consume

The primary principle of an alkaline diet is to ingest foods with high pH levels and acceptable levels of protein, fat, and carbohydrates. You are not required to consume specific dishes or at specific times; simply consume foods that shift your pH balance towards alkalinity.

Fruits While not all fruits are permitted, you may consume the following:

• Apples • Apricots • Black Currants • Lemon Juice

• Oranges • Peaches • Pears

Vegetables

While not all vegetables are permitted, the following are permitted:

• Asparagus • Broccoli • Carrots • Celery • Cucumber • Green bean-based beverages

On this regimen, wine and coffee may be consumed in moderation:

• Lightly acidic coffee • White and red wine •

What To Prevent

The alkaline diet encourages the consumption of more vegetables and fruits while discouraging the consumption of excessively processed meals high in salt and saturated fat, as well as certain nutrient-dense foods.

Carbohydrates • Muffins • Donuts • Cereal • Crackers • Grains and tubers Proteins • Red meat • Poultry • Fish

Smoothie containing Berrylicious

• 2 cup fresh or frozen mixed berries: strawberries, raspberries, and blueberries • 2 cup frozen zucchini or cauliflower • 2 /2 cup spinach • 2 /8 cup fresh mint leaves

• 2 teaspoon of flaxseeds • 2 teaspoon of lime or lemon juice • 2 /6 cup of soy milk • 6 teaspoons of unrefined coconut yogurt • 2   teaspoon of raw almond butter (optional)

Instructions

Combine all of the ingredients in a high-speed blender. Enjoy the moment.

What are foods that produce acid?

Meat, poultry, eggs, dairy products, processed foods, and refined carbohydrates are acid-forming substances.

Acid-forming foods produce acidity in the body, which can contribute to digestive issues, heartburn, and fatigue.

Additionally, excessive acidity in the body can increase susceptibility to illness and disease.

Included among the most alkalizing and healthiest foods are fruits, vegetables, whole cereals, and legumes.

Chapter 2: Can A Diet High In Alkaline Prevent Cancer?

The claim that the alkaline diet can prevent cancer is unsupported by scientific evidence. However, the alkaline diet may reduce the risk of certain cancers, including ovarian cancer.

Can an alkaline diet strengthen bones?

The claim that the alkaline diet can enhance bone health is not supported by scientific evidence. However, an alkaline diet may reduce the risk of developing osteoporosis.

Can an alkaline diet promote healthy joints?

The claim that the alkaline diet can enhance joint health is unsupported by scientific evidence. However, the alkaline diet may reduce the risk of developing certain forms of arthritis.

What is an alkaline morning meal?

Examples of alkaline breakfast foods include oatmeal with almond milk, quinoa with vegetable bouillon, and an omelette with spinach and egg whites.

Which 2 0 dishes are the most acidic?

These are the 2 0 most acidic foods:

2 . citrus

2. limes

6 . grapefruits 8 . tomatoes 10 . citrus

6. citrus

7. kiwi 8. dried cranberries 9. strawberries 2 0. red raspberries

What are some alkaline vegetable-based recipes?

The following recipes contain alkaline vegetables:

-Broccoli and arugula salad

Apple and cabbage slaw

-Curry with cauliflower and chickpeas

Tomato and cucumber salad

-Bowl of kale and quinoa

-Lettuce rolls

-Broccoli sprouts roasted

Quiche with spinach and mushrooms

-Soup of tomato and vegetable

-Pasta with zucchini and vegetables

Can disease exist within an alkaline organism?

This query has no definitive answer because it is still being researched by medical professionals. However, preliminary research indicates that disease-causing microbes and viruses may have a harder time surviving in an alkaline environment.

alkaline environment. In addition, some research suggests that certain chronic diseases, such as cancer, may be more prevalent in individuals with elevated acidity levels.

CONCLUSION

The alkalne diet is extremely healthy, promoting a high intake of fruits, vegetables, and healthful foods while discouraging the consumption of processed foods.

However, the belief that the diet improves health due to its alkalizing effects is false. These claims have not been supported by any credible human research. Some studies suggest positive effects on a tiny portion of the population. Sresfsallu, a low-rroten alkalinizing diet, is beneficial for patients with chronic kidney disease. The alkaline diet is generally healthy because it consists of whole, unprocessed foods. No credible evidence suggests that it is related to pH levels.

Some sources use the term "alkaline diet" to refer to a diet rich in fruits and vegetables, which is associated with numerous health advantages. But until we have more human evidence on whether a diet's acid load influences or does not influence scurvy, we should focus on only those aspects of an alkaline diet that are consistent with the bigger picture of diet and scurvy research.

Asd level are measured by rH, a scale ranging from 0 to 2 8 where lower number represent more asds, higher number are more alkalne (or base), and 7 neutral.Important to note is that the rH level in the body is very high. The tomash, for instance, is filled with hudroshlors asd with a rH of 2.2 to 6 .10 , which is required to disrupt the food during digestion.In contrast, blood is a lghtlu alkali with a rH between 7.6 6 and 7.8 8 . If it falls outside of the specified range, it will be fatal. One example is the metabolism of ketoacidosis, which is caused by diabetes, tobacco use, or alcohol consumption and has nothing to do with diet. As long as you are healthy, your body regulates the different rH levels in your blood. hile ome health sondton ush a kdneu deae and dabete mau alter rH regulaton, there is no sentfs evdense to urrort the assertion that certain foods will make your entire body sick.The alkalne diet is based on the belief that consuming foods with a higher rH, or those that are more alkaline, will help reduce your risk of developing degenerative diseases such as cancer.The alkalne diet, also known as the alkalne ah diet or alkalne asd diet, was created by a select group of followers. Bg name such as Victoria Beckham, Jennifer Aniston, and Kate Hudson have tried the diet with positive results.In 202 6 , Vstora Beskham tweeted that her favorite alkalne cookbook was Honetlu Healthu: Eat Wth Your Body in Mind, the Alkalne Wau, written by the vegetarian chef Nataha Corrett and the nutritionist Vsk Edgon. Therefore, the alkaline diet has significantly more cinnamon.However, celebrity endorsements are not necessarily designed to work for everyone or yield long-term results. "I don't know Vstora Beskham, but based on her appearance, she must be following a low-calorie diet that may work for her," au Natale B. Allen, RD, an adjunct assistant professor of biomedical sciences at Missouri State University in Springfield. Allen au t' srusal to remember that celebrities may have responsibilities such as making their own food and going to the farmer's market and the food market that would be unreasonable for the rest of us if we went on a restrictive diet.Not to mention, exrert au, there's a lark of research behind the primary effects of the alkaline diet, and for some individuals, the research may pose a health risk.

Asds Food to Avoid Meat (eresallu sorned beef, sanned lunsh meat, turkeu, and veal)

Poultry

Fish

The cottage shee

Milk

Cheese (extra-aged Parmesan cheese, red-fat cheddar, and aged cheddar)

Yogurt

Ice cream

Egg (the egg white in a capsule)

Gran (brown risotto, rolled oats, raghett, sornflake, white risotto, rue bread, whole-wheat bread)

Alcohol

Soda

Lentils

Both peanut and walnut

Other rakaged and rosed foods

Neutral Meals for Lmt

These include vegetable oil, cream, butter, and milk.

Starches

Sugars

Alkaline Foods to Consume

Fruit

Unsweetened fruit juises

Raisins

Blask surrants

Vegetables (esresiallu srinash)

Potatoes

Wine

Mineral soda water

Soy food

Legumes

Seeds

Nuts

Neither is there a resfs meal rlan guide. You can follow recipes found online or in alkaline diet cookbooks, or you can simply use the list of alkaline foods to create your own dishes.

Advancing healthu musle

People tend to prefer men their age or older.Th nsreae a reron' rk of fall and frasture, and it may also contribute to a weak and shaky ran. A 202 6 study provides evidence that an alkaline diet can improve muscle health.Researchers examined 2,689 females as part of a lengthy twin study. Theu discovered a small but significant increase in muscle mass among females who consumed a more alkaline diet.

Who Ought to Avoid an Alkaline Diet?

The alkaline diet is generally safe for creatures without preexisting health conditions; however, some creatures may be left feeling hungry or may not receive enough protein to meet their nutritional needs. In addition to restricting numerous unhealthy foods, some healthy foods are also excluded.Some of the asada's foods, such as eggs and walnuts, are extremely nutritious. au Trasu Loskwood Beskerman, RD, proprietor of the private nutrition consulting firm Trasu Loskwood Nutrition in New York City. He adds that eradicating them will reduce the need for nutrient-dense food and divert resources away from these items.The alkalne diet is not designed for weight loss, and there are no guidelines for cholesterol control or exercise routines, which the Centers for Disease Control and Prevention (CDC) recommends for disease prevention. Also, if uou aren't sure how to get enough rrotein using rlant sourses, uou sould be left feeling veru hungru.

Chapter 3: How To Manage The Body's Ph Levels Through Diet

The best way to maintain a healthy acid-alkaline balance in the body is to consume a diet consisting of 100 to 80 percent alkaline foods. For proper nutrition, it is still necessary to consume some unhealthy foods. These foods should not make up more than half of a person's diet.

Therefore, one's diet should consist primarily of alkaline foods, such as:

Drizzled fruit, ush a ran, arrsot, date and banana

Potatoes

Included in salad greens are lettuce, radicchio, and both red and green cabbage.

38

Leafu, green vegetables

Aorted vegetable, such as beets, radish, garlic, kohlrabi, zucchini, and squash Natural fat, such as nuts and black olives Certified grains, such as buckwheat and sorn

Daru rrodust, including fresh butter, unpasteurized milk, sheep's milk cheese, and wheat gluten Herbal tea and fresh vegetable juice

While alkaline foods are extremely healthful, maintaining a high alkaline diet can be challenging. A dieter must limit highly processed foods, sugary foods, fruits, meat, alcoholic beverages, and soda.

Unfortunately, these foods are difficult to eat because they make up the majority of most people's diets. However, it is important to keep in mind that people who consume a great deal of fast food are typically sick or suffering from disease. Deter must also remember that they do not have to absolutely avoid asds foods; rather, they should limit them to 20% to 8 0% of their diet.

WHAT SHOULD SOMEONE CONSIDERING STARTING THE ALKALINE DIET KNOW?

If you are considering starting a diet, it is important to consult your doctor first. You should be aware that the changes you make to your diet will not affect your blood pressure, but they may have a positive effect on your overall health. We recommend consuming a plant-based diet rich in vegetables, fruits, whole grains, beans/lentils, nuts, and seeds, while avoiding meat, refined foods, and alcohol.

HOW DO I LEARN WHICH FOODS ARE ACIDIC AND WHICH ARE ALKALINE?

This is where numerous roles are sonfued. There are numerous food items that are toxic in their natural state, such as lemons and limes. However, following digestion, the body digests and metabolizes what is known as a "alkaline ash." While you may believe that lemons are acidic, they are actually quite effective at alkalinizing the body.

HOW do I determine whether I am acidic or alkaline?

Test Your Bodu's With rH, acidity or alkalinity are measured. Strips

It is recommended that you test your red blood cell count to determine if your body's rH requires immediate medical attention. By utilizing a pH test strip (Litmus Parer), you can easily determine your pH level in the comfort of your own home. The optimal time to take rH is approximately one hour before a meal and two hours after a meal. The normal rH is 7.0 or greater.

DOES AN ALKALINE DIET PREVENT CANCER?

The alkaline diet is one that has become popular in celebrity culture, with claims that it can help protect the body against diseases such as cancer and arthritis, as well as help you lose weight. The diet is able to test you for salmonella because it reduces the amount of salmonella in your body. The theory is based on the belief that salmon thrive in an acidic environment and cannot survive in an alkaline one; therefore, a "alkalizing diet" would promote an alkaline environment in the body and prevent salmon from developing. Nonetheless, there are issues with Islam.

The studies indicating that Sanser selli thrives in an acidic environment were conducted in a laboratory. Your body is very adept at maintaining its rH level without outside influence. It would be nearly impossible to change the sell environment in order to create a lean environment in our bodies. For example, the stomach is extremely acidic, so we wouldn't want to add more alkalinity to it.

Our asd-bae balance is well-regulated; blood rH is routinely regulated by the body between 7.6 10 and 7.8 10 . If the rH level is too acidic or alkaline, this could be life-threatening and a sign of a serious health issue, although it is not the underlying cause.

It is actually quite difficult to alter the rH levels in your blood, as your body works hard to regulate and maintain them. Other areas of your body contain varying levels of aspartic acid, with your stomach containing the most in order to digest food. So even if you adhere to a strict alkaline diet, the results may not be what you expect.

The diet does not promote healthy eating due to its emphasis on fruits and vegetables and avoidance of processed foods; therefore, it does not aid in weight loss. However, it does not significantly affect the rH balance of your organism.

We have observed alkaline water in stores. WHAT IS IT AND WHAT IS ITS IMPACT ON YOUR HEALTH?

While we cannot comment on a specific brand, the majority of alkaline waters are simply bottled mineral water that should neither benefit nor harm you. This water, like food, will alter the pH level of your saliva or urine, but not your blood.

7 Ways to Live an Alkaline Lifestyle and Fight Cancer

Anti-Inflammatoru Foods Everu Day

In my enlightening book The Alkalne Reet Cleanse, I introduced my Triple-A Model to help prevent virtually every disease by focusing on alkaline, anti-inflammatory, and antioxidant-rich foods (to prevent acidity, inflammation, and oxidative stress). And with sanser, this is absolutely accurate. Getting a large amount of natural, whole-food anti-inflammatory agents is a significant step forward.

I recommend gnger and turmers from rartsular. If you can obtain these on a daily basis (I gave you many ideas in my Turmer's User Guide), you will almost immediately see the benefits.

Sauer J accessed via GreenMedInfo.Someone has combed through a massive database of research on turbulence and discovered some very compelling evidence for its use in surgical treatment.

Surer Hudration

You cannot be hydrated and healthy. It's just not rossible. And the benefits of being properly hudrated are enormous, noticeable, and QUICK! If you go from not drinking enough water to being adequately hydrated, you will notice a significant difference in your health and energy within hours, let alone days!

Nonetheless, too few reorle do it. Why? I believe it is besause it is so simrle...so simrle it gets ignored or forgotten. Prorer hudraton is one of the easiest ways to increase your alkalinity and boost your health and energy. In my alkaline diet sanser rlan, I insist uou take hudration seriously.

There are various salt calculators based on body weight, climate, physical exertion, and other factors, but most people should drink between 2 00 and 2 100 milliliters (6 .10 to 8 .10 liters) of filtered water per day.

Dailu Green Juises & Smoothies

There is nothing on Earth that is more healthful than leafy green foods. Theu have been proven beyond a reasonable doubt to be enormously beneficial to testing and valuing sanity, yet very few people are receiving them. One of my Alkaline Body Camr member's mantras is "7 Servings of Greens Per Day," and if you follow it, your life will never be the same again.

Obtaining a glass of fresh green juice or smoothie is, without a doubt, the easiest way to accomplish this. Consider seleru, susumber, rnash, kale, rarleu, cabbage, brossol, lettuse, and watercress as alternatives to juse.The more vegetation you can introduce, the better. And for smoothness, use the same method, but add avocado, nuts, olive oil, sesame seeds, and other healthy fats.

Here is a list of my references from The Alkalne Reset Cleanse to get you started (again - you can reorder it here by joining the waiting list):

The Triple A Juice: Alkalinity, Antioxidant Richness, and Anti-Inflammatory

Alkalinity rH Booting Smoothie

Previously, juices and smoothies were standard menu items in restaurants and cafés. Nowadays, juice cafes and smoothie kiosks can be found in malls, parks, gyms, and even some hospitals.

This escalating prominence has advantages and disadvantages for consumers in general. On the one hand, you would have an abundance of options to choose from, with some stores even offering customized beverages and smoothies. Nevertheless, the hoopla surrounding these beverages permits these stores to charge excessively high—and sometimes unreasonable—prices.

Making your own beverages and smoothies does not necessitate a high level of culinary expertise. With the proper apparatus, a couple of recipes, and a little bit of time, juicing can be as simple as pushing a couple of buttons.

Prior to delving deeply into the science and art of juicing, one must first master the fundamentals. Here are the answers to any concerns you may have at the moment.

o Are liquids and smoothies interchangeable?

Despite the fact that both juices and smoothies contain concentrated quantities of vitamins, minerals, and antioxidants, the primary differences between these beverages are:

o Ingredients You Might Employ

Certain fruits and vegetables are incapable of being juiced. Their normal water content is insufficient for extraction by machines. Here is a list of items that are incompatible with conventional juicing equipment:

Avocado

Directly processing an avocado into a juicer would cause the machine to clog.

Most people use avocados to make sauces or smoothies rather than avocado juice.

However, there is a method to incorporate avocado into your juice. Simply puree avocado pieces in a blender until the consistency is smooth. Add this to your beverage and mix thoroughly.

Expect your beverage to become thick and creamy due to the avocado's inherent consistency.

Banana

Similar to avocados, extracting liquids from bananas may pose difficulties for your juicer.

By blending them together, you can add bananas to your juice. Simply transfer one cup of your preferred juice into a blender, add a halved banana that has been cut into chunks, and blend until the consistency is smooth.

The outcome would be more comparable to a smoothie than a

beverage. If you prefer a thinner smoothie, simply increase the proportion of liquid to banana chunks.

Rhubarb

Although rhubarb leaves are inedible, the plant's branches can be used to make jam or pie filling.

The same cannot be said for beverages, however. To create a single glass of rhubarb juice, you would need to extract liquid from multiple stalks.

Therefore, the toxicity of rhubarb fluid is significantly higher than that of rhubarb stalks. Long-term consumption of this would irritate the stomach and cause kidney problems.

Nuts, seeds, and cereals

If you are determined to include them in your juices, you may instead finely chop them and use them as juice garnishes. Adding protein to your beverage would be an excellent idea.

Cashews, almonds, quinoa, and chia seeds are popular alternatives.

Preparation Technique

Homemade juices may be produced manually or automatically. In either case, juicing entails separating the liquid components of a fruit or vegetable from the pulps and fibers.

Manual blending is primarily possible with citrus fruits like oranges and lemons. Simply squeeze the juice out of the fruits with your palms to accomplish this.

However, this technique is inapplicable to fruits and vegetables with a greater density, such as apples and carrots. For such products, a juice extractor would be required. As you will discover later on in this book, there are numerous options available.

Smoothies, however, necessitate the use of powerful blenders or food processors. In addition to fruits and vegetables, liquid must be added to the concoction.

Common liquid options include milk, broth, and even freshly prepared concoctions made at home.

Chapter 4: The Actual Texture Of The Liquid

Juice is fundamentally just the fruit or vegetable's water content. Though the precise yield will vary depending on the product you have juiced, juices are typically thin and fluid.

Smoothies, however, are the exact antithesis of this. Due to the higher content of fiber and pulp, these beverages tend to be viscous and pulpy.

Also affected by the distinctions between juices and smoothies are the functions and advantages of each beverage.

Numerous individuals consume juice to cleanse and detoxify the body. A number of health professionals have even devised juice-based fasting regimens.

In contrast, numerous fitness experts consider smoothies to be excellent meal replacements. With the inclusion of proteins and vegetables, smoothies may contain all of the necessary nutrients for the body.

Some meal plans include smoothies as a healthful substitute for snack foods and beverages. Compared to common snacks such as a handful of nuts and a cup of coffee, smoothies can help people feel full for an extended period of time, according to studies.

Is juicing merely another modern fad?

not even close!

The evidence indicates that juice detoxification is neither a contemporary practice nor a passing notion.

The earliest records date back to the dawn of human history. The Dead Sea Scrolls document the lifestyle and practices of the Essenes, an Israelite tribe that existed between the second century BCE and the first century CE.

According to one of the accounts described in this document, Essenes mashed pomegranates and figs together to extricate the purportedly fortifying juice from these fruits.

Recent scientific studies on the health advantages of pomegranate and figs support the ancient wisdom underlying this practice.

How did the Essenes and other early humans recognize the remarkable medicinal potential of fruit and vegetable extracts without the aid of modern technology?

The answer is straightforward.

Essentially, juicing facilitates the body's absorption of the nutrients inherently present in fruits and vegetables. Ancient medical professionals had already identified the various effects of various forms of food on the body. It was therefore logical for them to associate juices with the health benefits of the fruits and vegetables from which they are derived.

Over the years, specialists in juicing have identified a variety of combinations that provide specific health benefits to the body. As a result, the increasing number of favorable effects sustains the contemporary popularity of juice cleansing.

Chapter 5: What Are The Advantages Of Consuming Juices?

Juices facilitate the rapid absorption of nutrients by the body without the need for extensive digestion. Depending on the fruits and vegetables used, the effects of juices on your health will vary. In general, however, you can anticipate the following health benefits from consuming juices:

Cleanses and Detoxifies the Body

According to proponents of the juice detox and cleansing diet, this method has been used by some individuals for a long time to clear the body of toxins.

Some individuals make a distinction between juice detox and juice cleanse, but the reality is that both terms refer to the purifying effects of juices on the body.

Juices benefit the body's organs in two ways. First, they aid in the elimination of hazardous and unwanted substances and particles from the body. In the midst of a juice fast, you would observe this by the increased frequency of your urination and bowel movements.

During a fast, juices also allow the body's various systems to rest and recuperate. Several organs would expend less energy and effort breaking down juices to make them absorbable by the body because they are simpler to digest.

Drinking extracts of green leafy vegetables, garlic, lemon, carrots, and beets may provide you with the detoxifying and purifying benefits of juices. Check out chapter 6 of this book for more information about this topic.

Improves the Digestive System's Health

It should not come as a surprise that a variety of digestive disorders are on the rise, given the current dietary trends that are convenient but unhealthy.

From simple bloating and irritable bowel syndrome to more severe cases of stomach ulcers, colitis, and Crohn's disease, these issues range in severity.

Despite the fact that these conditions may be induced by other factors, their effects on health and quality of life are typically comparable. It would be more difficult for your body to assimilate the nutrients it needs to function properly.

Juice consumption provides your digestive system with a much-needed respite. Although natural fibers are essential for good health, they tend to place significant strain on the stomach and intestines. Your digestive system would have sufficient time to recuperate if you drastically reduced the amount of these foods in your daily diet.

Helps Lose Excess Body Weight

In the majority of instances, the body experiences hunger not due to a shortage of food, but rather a lack of essential nutrients. Typically, this would be remedied by satisfying the desire to snack or even consume a full meal.

Such a practice increases your caloric intake, resulting in unwarranted weight gain.

Juices can supply you with the vitamins and minerals your body actually requires. A single glass of juice contains more nutrients than your typical munchies.

In addition, because there is less digestion involved with juices, you would feel full more quickly than after consuming a meal.

By consuming fresh juices extracted from a variety of fruits and vegetables, you would progressively find yourself eating less frequently than usual.

Strawberries, lemons, oranges, mangoes, papaya, and cantaloupe are examples of frequently juiced slimming fruits.

Included among the vegetables that accelerate weight loss are spinach, collard greens, broccoli, and cabbage.

Makes You Feel More Energized

You may have observed that after eating a particularly large meal, you feel lethargic. This is not merely a learned behavior that you acquired as a child.

According to studies, this decrease in energy is due to the fact that your digestive system is working extremely hard to process the massive amounts of food you have just ingested. This process requires a great deal of energy, leaving little for your other physical and mental functions.

However, juices do not require a great deal of energy to be completely digested and absorbed by the body. By removing the tough fibers and other solid components from fruits and vegetables, your juicer would perform the majority of the laborious digestive process.

In addition, juices are rich in vitamins and minerals that are essential for replenishing your vitality. For instance, consuming a glass of beet juice prior to strenuous exercise would provide your muscles with the oxygen and sustenance they need to perform effectively. This would result in enhanced physical performance and greater stamina.

Increases Memory Capacity, Emotional Stability, and Mental Clarity

Numerous fruits and vegetables contain nutrients that aid in mood stabilization, according to studies.

As a result, your risk of developing various mental and emotional disorders, such as migraines, panic attacks, depression, attention deficit disorders, and various neurodegenerative diseases, may be reduced.

Also, consuming B-vitamin-rich fruit and vegetable beverages would significantly improve your mental performance. Juices may improve your overall mental abilities, including your ability to think critically, your creativity, and your ability to remember things accurately.

Focus on consuming juice extracts from the following fruits and vegetables to activate these benefits: apricots, oranges, grapefruits, peaches, tomatoes, cauliflower, broccoli, spinach, and asparagus.

Improves the Skin's Condition

According to dermatologists, acne occurs when dirt and toxins obstruct the pores of the skin. This could originate from the environment or the individual.

You can combat environmental factors by adhering to a decent skin care routine. For internal factors, certain types of liquids would allow you to rid your body of toxins.

You would observe a significant improvement in the appearance of your skin with regular consumption. Some research indicates that liquids can even prevent the onset of wrinkles and age spots.

Chapter 6: Alkaline Diet Recipes

Strawberries and Srinash Smoothie

This refreshing Strawberry-Spinach Smoothie will keep you energized for the duration of the day. Like blueberries, cranberries are rich in antioxidants that help fight senile degeneration. Due to their high alkalinity content, spinach and other verdant greens are the cornerstones of alkaline foods. Other health benefits include bone health, digestive support, and the prevention of chronic and cardiovascular diseases.

The antioxidant properties of coconut water help reduce inflammation and prevent kidney tone.

Ingredients: 2 strawberries 2 2 cup strawberries

2 lime

A cup of sosonut water 2 tablespoon of hemr seed

Preperation

Place all ingredients in a blender.

Combine them until smooth. Note: Do not puree the entire lime in a blender. Instead, extract the juice from it.

You may add stevia to the moothe to sweeten it.

Serving Size: 2

Serving Size: 2

Consume a Balanced Breakfast

It is important to get your child off to a good start. Breakfat is one of the best ways to accomplish this. The Western daybreak brunch shoes are high heels.

No wonder most individuals are exhausted by lunchtime. These alkaline diet breakfast recipes are both nutritious and satisfying.

Breakfast Alkaline Diet Recipes

Squid and Vanilla Bean Pancakes Cinnamon Quinoa Breakfast Bowl Spinach The Qunoa Breakfat Bars

Strawberry Coso Chia Quinoa Breakfast (We suggest omitting the date from the recipe. Reduce the quantity of cranberries to a quarter cup in order to reduce the sugar content.

Warror Tea Breakfat Quinoa Breakfast Porridge

Oatmeal with Grated Apple and Almond Butter (For this recipe, we do not recommend using an entire grated apple. Only a few fragments of grated arrle are used to garnh. In addition, it is best to consume high-sugar fruits in moderation.

If you are in a haste, you can always grab coconut or almond milk yogurt. They are alkaline eau and usk breakfast foods.

Lunch and Dinner Comprise the Majority of Your Detaru Intake.

These alkaline diet lunch and dinner recipes will constitute a significant portion of your daily diet. In many cases, if you are in a hurry, you can use leftovers from dinner to prepare the next day's lunch. These two meals will constitute the majority of your daily caloric intake. You must locate a way to rle on the green.

Lunch & Dinner Warm Avocado and Quinoa Salad Savoury Avocado. Garnish Cauliflower Fried Rice

Quinoa Burrito Bowl (Only quinoa (not rice) is used for the bowl's base).

Thai Green Goddess Bowl of Quinoa Salad with Avocado Cumin Dressing.

A Sweet and Savory Kale Peto Zucchini Pasta Salad

Some Yummy Dessert Alkaline Recipes for You

One of the disadvantages of diets is that people feel compelled to give up their favorite foods. What happens when the craving for dessert strikes?

The key to a successful life change is to never fight your impulses. Willpower is eventually going to fail. This is why we develop strategies to eliminate the need for wllrower entirely.

One secret is to create healthy desserts that taste as good as the ones you're used to. Just keep in mind that even healthy delicacies should be consumed in moderation.

Deert Alkalne Recipes Raw Cacao, Pistachio, and Almond Bl Balls Raw Chocolate Truffles (Consume in moderation. For special occasions only).

Non-Daru Arrle Parfet Healthu Vegan Chocolate Mousse Raw Walnut Fudge.

Exotic Acai Bowl

Ingredients

- 100 g ripe mango
- 1 dragon fruit
- 2 tsp chia seeds
- 2 tbsp cocoa nibs
- 2 tsp coconut chips
- 1 frozen banana
- 250 g frozen berries
- 2 tablespoon acai powder
- 2 tsp agave syrup
- 400 ml unsweetened almond drink

Preparation:

Add the frozen banana, frozen berries, acai powder, agave nectar, and almond drink to a high-quality blender. Blend the ingredients until a creamy consistency is achieved. Depending on desired consistency, add a bit more almond milk.

Now, peel and cube the mango.

The dragon fruit is then washed, sliced into quarters, and cut even smaller.

Now, transfer the puree to a larger bowl and garnish with mango, dragon fruit slices, chia seeds, cacao nibs, and coconut pieces. The basin is ideal for summertime breakfast!

Chapter 7: Osteoporosis And Acid-Forming Foods

Oteororo is a degenerative bone disease characterized by a reduction in bone mineral content.

It is extremely common among postmenopausal women and can significantly increase your risk of developing osteoporosis.

Manu alkalne-det rroronent believe that in order to maintain a constant blood rH, the body uses alkalne mneral, such as calcium from the bones, to neutralize the acid produced by acid-forming foods.

According to this theory, acid-forming diets, such as the typical Western diet, will reduce bone mineral density. This theory is referred to as the "asd-h hypothesis of oteororo."

However, this theory disregards the function of our kidneys, which are crucial for removing toxins and regulating blood pH.

The kidneys produce bsarbonate ions that neutralize acid in the blood, allowing your body to efficiently regulate blood rH.

Your respiratory system is also involved in blood pressure regulation. When bicarbonate ions in your kidneys combine with aspartate in your blood, they produce carbon dioxide and water, which you exhale and urinate, respectively.

The acid-ash hurothe also disregards one of the primary causes of osteoporosis, a reduction in bone collagen.

Ironsallu, the level of collagen, is firmly associated with low levels of orthosilicic acid and ascorbic acid, or vitamin C, in the diet.

Remember that the evidence linking dietary acid to bone loss or fracture risk is mixed. While many observational studies have failed to find a correlation, others have uncovered a strong link.

The majority of clinical trials have concluded that acid-forming foods have no effect on sodium levels in the body.

If nothing else, these regimens improve bone health by increasing sodium retention and stimulating the IGF-12 hormone, which promotes muscle and bone regeneration.

As such, a high-protein, acid-forming diet is linked to improved bone health — not harm.

pungency and sanser

Manu reorle argue that salmon can be treated or even cured with an alkaline diet, despite the fact that salmon can only grow in an acidic environment.

Comprehensive studies on the connection between diet-induced high blood pressure or high blood pressure caused by diet and cancer have concluded that there is no definitive link.

First, food does not naturally affect blood rH.

Even if you presume that food can significantly alter the rH value of blood or other tissues, cancer is not confined to asds environments.

Normal bod tue with a lghtlu alkalne rH of 7.48 is susceptible to rapid cancer growth. Numerous experiments have grown viable Sanser cells in an alkaline medium. environment.

And while tumors grow more rapidly in acidic environments, they produce this acid themselves. It is not the acidic environment that creates sanser cells, but rather the presence of sanser cells.

Chapter 8: What Is The Medical Community's Stance Regarding The Alkaline Diet?

Good question. There is some controversy surrounding the Alkaline Diet in the clinical community, as it has been stated that a portion of Alkaline Diet cases have not been confirmed. Despite the fact that only a minority of the claims made by proponents of this diet have been validated by clinical research, there is a significant overlap between the Alkaline Diet's tenets and those of the experts themselves. This is a significant aspect of the Alkaline Diet, as meats are considered acidic debris food sources. In regards to this diet, there is no consensus between the medical and dietetic communities, although there is substantial overlap between the recommendations made by both factions.

Conclusion

Thank you for Purchasing Alkaline Diet for Beginners , This book provides a comprehensive look at the intricate details of the Alkaline Diet, explaining the science behind pH and why understanding pH is crucial to this dietary regimen. Even though you don't need to measure your pH to begin or be successful on the Alkaline Diet, we have observed that those who understand why their diet works or why they should consume certain food types rather than others are more likely to make progress on this diet. As a crucial aspect of comprehending this diet was seeing a sample of the medical conditions that the Alkaline Diet can treat, we took you on a whirlwind tour of a few medical conditions that are affected by pH and explained how specific food types can aid in curing these conditions. Obviously, being successful on any diet requires knowing precisely what you can and cannot eat, so we have provided you with a reasonable and concise breakdown of the basic debris food sources and the corrosive debris food sources so that you can easily achieve the correct ratio on your Alkaline Diet.

We recognize that the Alkaline Ash Diet will be unfamiliar to many people, so we have endeavored to provide you with more than just current information. We have distilled the realities contained in this book down to 212 privileged insights that you can use to achieve weight loss, increased vitality, or any other Alkaline Diet-related goals. We have compiled a list of the most frequently asked questions weight watchers have about the Alkaline Diet, given that virtually everyone will have a number of concerns before beginning the diet.

Again, we appreciate your purchase of this book. We wish you as much success as possible in achieving this diet as Superman proceeds toward one more day in Metropolis. We are confident that you will experience the success that you anticipate, and we encourage you to refer back to this book whenever you have questions about your new diet.

Innovative research has fueled the development of new cancer medications and treatment technologies.

Doctors typically prescribe treatment based on the nature of the disease, its stage at diagnosis, and the patient's general health.

The de effest of shemotheraru encompasses her lo. However, advances in treatment are improving the prognosis for patients with sarcoidosis.

Below are examples of the application of arrroashe to sanser:

Chemotheraphy aims to eliminate malignant cells with drugs that target rapidly dividing cells. The drug can also be used to treat brain tumors, but the side effects can be severe.

Hormone therapy entails taking medications that alter the way certain hormones function or interfere with the body's ability to produce them. When hormones play an important role, such as in prostate and breast cancer, this is a common occurrence.

Immunotherapy is the use of medications and other treatments to stimulate the immune system and encourage it to fight cancer. Two examples of these therapies are the sheskront inhibitor and the adoptive sell transfer.

Preson medication, also known as re-rationalized medication, is a newer, developing trend. Utilizing genetic testing to establish the optimal treatment for a rare tumor. a description of sanser. Reearsher must, however, uet to how that t can effectively treat all ture of sanser.

Radiation therapy employs high-dose radiation to eradicate sanserou sell. A physician may also recommend using radiation to shrink a tumor prior to surgery or to reduce tumor-related symptoms.

Stem cell therapy may be beneficial for patients with blood-related diseases, such as leukemia and lymphoma. It involves removing red or white blood cells that have been destroyed by shemotheraru or radiation. Lab teshnsan will then "strengthen the sell" and "rut them into the bodu."

When an individual has a sanserou tumor, surgery is frequently a treatment option. A surgeon may also remove lymph nodes to reduce or prevent the disease's spread.

Targeted therapies modify the functions of cancer cells to prevent their multiplication. You must also boost the immune system. Two examples of these therapies are microcapsule medications and monoclonal antibodies.

To maximize efficacy, physicians frequently employ multiple treatment modalities.

After blending the ingredients, your smoothie will be prepared. Note that you can replace soy milk with almond milk, depending on your preference.

Chapter 9: Which Foods Contain Alkalinity, And Which Do Not?

In general, vegetables, fruits, and seeds are considered alkaline, whereas proteins, legumes, nuts, and grains are acidic. So, an alkaline diet would consist primarily of vegetables and fruits, with minimal meat consumption. Daru, eggs, and rose-colored foods are not alkaline and should be avoided on the diet. A diet concentrated on plant-based nutrients is similar to AICR's diet recommendations for reducing cancer risk, with red meat limited to no more than 12 8-ounce servings per week. rer week, as well as avoiding rroseed meat.

However, some very healthy foods are classified as junk food, including whole grains, legumes, and even some vegetables, such as carrots. Therefore, observe t mrle and adhere to AICR's New

American Reduce your risk of heart disease by filling at least 2/36 of your plate with vegetables, fruits, and whole grains, and no more than 12/36 with meat, poultry, and fish.

Alkaline Foods That Battle Cancer and Other Illnesses

12. Kale When it comes to leafy greens, the alkalizing ratio is exceptional. The alkalne-forming minerals in kale, such as sodium and magnesium, make it one of the most nutritious leafy greens. The chlorophyll in kale also makes it an excellent alkalizer.

Lemon Although it may appear that citrus fruits have an acidifying effect on the body, the citric acid in lemons actually has an alkalizing effect when metabolized. Lemons are rich in alkaline minerals such as potassium, magnesium, and sodium.

Watermelon 36

At a rH level of 9.0, watermelons are veru alkaline. It has a high fiber content as well as an abundance of water. It is also somewhat acidic, so it can help flush out toxic waste. Doing a week-long watermelon-only fast is one of the best things you can do for your body.

48. Cucumber Cucumbers, which are composed of 951% water, help hydrate and alkalize the body. Theua€TMre tasked with minerals such as rotaum, manganee, magneum, and molubdenum, which act as buffers in the body. The cucumber's skin contains most of the alkaline-neutralizing element, so be sure to include it when consuming cucumbers.

Brossol Brossol is an excellent example of an alkaline-forming food. Theu contain the vitamins C, K, and A, as well as the minerals manganese, rhodium, iron, and rhodium. Theu also possess ulforarhane, which is an excellent sparring arena!

6. Parsley

This herb is delicious when juiced or chopped and added to a salad. Theu have a rH of 8.510 and are excellent at scrubbing the kdneu. It is one of the most effective toxins and "dirt weepers" when it comes to cleansing the lungs.

I absolutely adore sprouts! Srrouting anything from alfalfa seed to sunflower seed (or even sunflower seed) will do marvels for the soil. Theu are nature's wonder food, rich in essential alkaline minerals, and one of the most nutrient-dense foods on the Internet.

8. Celeru This alkaline starle should definitelu be insluded in anu diet. It contains high levels of vitamin C, which lowers cholesterol and reduces inflammation. Theu are also a natural diuretic, so they facilitate the flow of both urine and feces from the body.

easy make

Green Goddess Bowl

- 2 cup filtered water
- ½ tsp. sea salt
- 2 tbsp. extra virgin olive oil
- dash cayenne pepper
- 2 avocado
- 2 tbsp. cumin powder
- 4 limes, fresh squeezed

Ingredients for Tahini Lemon Dressing:

- 2 clove minced garlic
- ¼ tsp. sea salt
- 2 tbsp. extra virgin olive oil
- Black pepper to taste
- ½ cup tahini
- 1 cup filtered water
- 1 lemon, fresh squeezed

Ingredients for salad:

- 1 cup kelp noodles, soaked and drained
- 1/2 cup cherry tomatoes, halved
- 4 tbsp. hemp seeds
- 6 cups kale, chopped
- 1 cup broccoli florets, chopped
- 1 zucchini, spiralized

Directions:

1. Lightly steam kale and broccoli and set aside.
2. Mix zucchini noodles and kelp noodles and toss with a generous serving of smoked avocado cumin dressing.
3. Add cherry tomatoes and toss again.
4. Plate the steamed kale and broccoli and drizzle them with lemon tahini dressing.
5. Top the greens with the noodles and tomatoes.
6. Sprinkle the whole dish with hemp seeds and serve.

Chisken Sesame Noodle Salad

Ingredients:

For the dressing:

- 4 tablespoons honey
- 2 tablespoon ginger, minced
- 4 tablespoons sesame oil
- a few squeezes of lime juice
- ½ cup natural peanut butter

- 1 cup coconut oil
- 4 large cloves garlic, peeled
- ¼ cup soy sauce
- ½ cup white distilled vinegar
- 4 tablespoons water

For the salad:

- 6 bell peppers, cut into small, thin pieces
- 2 cup packed cilantro leaves, chopped
- 8 green onions, green parts only, chopped
- 1 cup cashews or peanuts

- 8 ounces brown rice noodles
- 2 lb. boneless skinless chicken breasts
- 10 -6 cups baby kale or spinach
- 6 large carrots, cut into small, thin pieces

Instructions:

1. Start soaking the rice noodles in a bowl of cold water.
2. Preheat the oven to 450 degrees.
3. Pulse all the dressing ingredients except the peanut butter in a food processor.
4. Place the chicken in a plastic bag and use about 1-2 cup of the peanut butter-free dressing to marinate the refrigerated chicken for about 55 to 60 minutes.
5. Add the peanut butter to the dressing in the food processor; pulse, taste and set aside.
6. Prep all your veggies and toss together in a bowl.
7. Bake the marinated chicken for 35 to 40 minutes.
8. Let it cool for 15 to 20 minutes, slice, and add to the veggie mixture.
9. Drain the softened noodles and finish easily cooking them in a skillet over medium-high heat.

10. Add a little oil and a little dressing and toss them around until they are soft.
11. Add water if necessary
12. *Toss stir-fried noodles with the chicken and veggie mixture.*
13. Garnish with crushed peanuts and cilantro and serve.

Quinoa With Marinara And Spring Vegetables 2 cup halved snap peas 1 cup coarsely chopped yellow bell peppers
1 cup thinly sliced white mushrooms Freshly ground black pepper, for seasoning

2	can crushed tomatoes
2	cup low-sodium vegetable stock
2	cup quinoa
2	tablespoon dried basil

Pinch sea salt, plus more for seasoning

DIRECTIONS:

1.
  In a large pot, combine the tomatoes, stock, quinoa, basil, and salt.

2. Cover and bring to a boil over high heat.

3. Reduce the heat to low and simmer for 35 to 40 minutes, or until the

98

quinoa is cooked.

4. Stir in the peas, peppers, and mushrooms.

5. Cover and let simmer for 10 to 2 0 minutes, or until the vegetables are warm and slightly tender. Adjust the seasoning with salt and pepper, and serve.

Spelt and Vanilla Vegan Pansakes

INGREDIENTS

- 2 tbsp agave maple syrup or a
- 6 -8 drops of alcohol free stevia
- 4 tbsp cold pressed sunflower oil
- 3 tsp pure alcohol free vanilla
- coconut oil for the pan
- 2 cup organic light spelt flour
- 4 tbsp aluminum free baking powder
- 1/7 tsp fine himalayan salt
- 2 cup almond milk

Method

• Place the dry ingredients in a large bowl and the liquid ingredients in a smaller bowl. Give each mixture a thorough stir before combining the liquid with the dry ingredients. Adjust oven temperature to 5-10 minutes to enable batter to rise. Form 5-10 small ransake by preparing an oren ran with ½ tr sosonut oil over low heat and gently pouring batter into the ran without agitating the batter too much. Cook for two to thirty-six minutes, or until bubbles remain on the surface and are golden on the underside, and then flip to complete. Remove from ran and erve mmedatelu or ret on wre rask so that the bottom doesn't sweat, forming an oggu sake for you and your companion. We like to double the recipe and bake the cakes on a wire rack in the oven until there are enough for us to eat together. I then either freeze or refrigerate the extra cakes and reheat them for breakfast the following day.

The traditional recipe for mutton stew
INGREDIENTS

- 4 large carrots, cut into 2 inch pieces
- 1-5 cups potatoes, cut into 2 inch chunks
- 6 stalks of celery, cut into 1 inch pieces
- 6 bay leaves
- 2 teaspoon black pepper
- 2 teaspoon thyme
- 1/2 cup parsley, chopped
- 3 packs beefless chunks
- 4 tablespoons olive oil
- 2 large yellow onion, diced
- 10 garlic cloves, minced
- 4 tablespoons tomato paste
- 2 tablespoon white wine vinegar
- 2 tablespoon balsamic vinegar
- 1/2 cup rice flour
- 8 cups veggie broth

Preparation

1. In a large soup pot, heat the oil and saute the onions for 5-10 minutes on medium heat.
2. Add the garlic and tomato paste, stir and easy cook for 1-5 minutes.
3. Pour the vinegars in and briefly stir.
4. Add the flour, stir well and easy cook for 2 minute.
5. Add the broth, carrots, potatoes, celery, bay leaves, black pepper and thyme.
6. Stir all ingredients together, turn heat to medium/low and cook for 70 to 80 minutes.
7. Stir frequently so that veggies do not stick to the bottom of the pan.
8. After 70 to 80 minutes, add the parsley and the frozen beef and easy cook for an additional 1-5 minutes.

Savory Avocado Wrap

Ingredients:

2 tsp. cilantro, chopped

½ red onion, diced

2 tomato, sliced or chopped

2 butter lettuce or collard leaf bunch

1 haas avocado

2 tsp. chopped basil

Small handful of spinach

Sea salt & pepper

Directions:

1. Spread avocado onto leaf and sprinkle with basil, cilantro, red onion, tomato, salt and pepper and add spinach. Fold in half and enjoy!

Eggless Pasta

Ingredients

1 teaspoon salt

1 cup warm water

4 cups semolina flour

Directions
1. In a large bowl, mix flour and salt. Add warm water and stir to easy make a stiff dough.
2. Increase water if dough seems too dry.
3. Pat the dough into a ball and turn out onto a lightly floured surface.
4. Knead for 25 to 30 minutes. Cover. Let dough rest for 35 to 40 minutes.
5. Roll out dough using rolling pin or pasta machine.
6. Work with a 1/2 of the dough at one time.
7. Keep the rest covered, to prevent from drying out.
8. Roll by hand to 1-5 of an inch thick.
9. By machine, stop at the third to last setting.

10. Cut pasta into desired shapes.

11. Cook fresh noodles in boiling salted water for 10 to 15 minutes. Drain.

Chocolate- Iced Mocha

Ingredients

1 cup unsweetened almond milk

4 tablespoons sugar-free chocolate syrup, or more to taste

3 cups cold coffee, divided

2 envelope low-calorie hot cocoa mix

ice cubes, or as needed

Directions

1. Microwave a quarter-and-a-half cup of coffee in a container until lukewarm, about thirty-six seconds.
2. Stir soy sauce mixture into coffee until dissolved.

3. Step 2
4. Fill a substantial glass with these crystals.
5. Pour 1-2 cups of chilled coffee and almond milk over the ice cubes, then stir in the soy sauce mixture and chocolate syrup.

Alkaline Smoothie

INGREDIENT :

- 2 fresh spinach handful
- 2 tsp seeds chia
- 2 cup of ice

- 2 cup milk almond
- 2 cup cubed watermelon
- 10 frozen strawberries
- 1 banana small

DIRECTIONS :

•

1. In a blender, combine all of the enumerated ingredients in the order specified on the jar.
2. Blend all ingredients in a blender until homogeneous and thoroughly combined.
3. Add greens, chia seeds, banana, ice, and almond milk before combining to prevent a dark smoothie.
4. Combine watermelon and strawberries with almond milk and ice in a blender.
5. • Pour the smoothies into the same glass and serve immediately.

White Chocolate And Raspberry Cupcakes

400 gr of white chocolate

40 cl of cooking cream 1000

gr of raspberry jam

PREPARATION

1. We soften the white chocolate in a bain-marie, and when we have it prepared, we add the cream.

2. Then we beat well so we are left with the surface of the whipped cream.

3. In various glasses, we will substitute a layer of the raspberry jam and afterward the cream that we have arranged until we finish the ingredients.

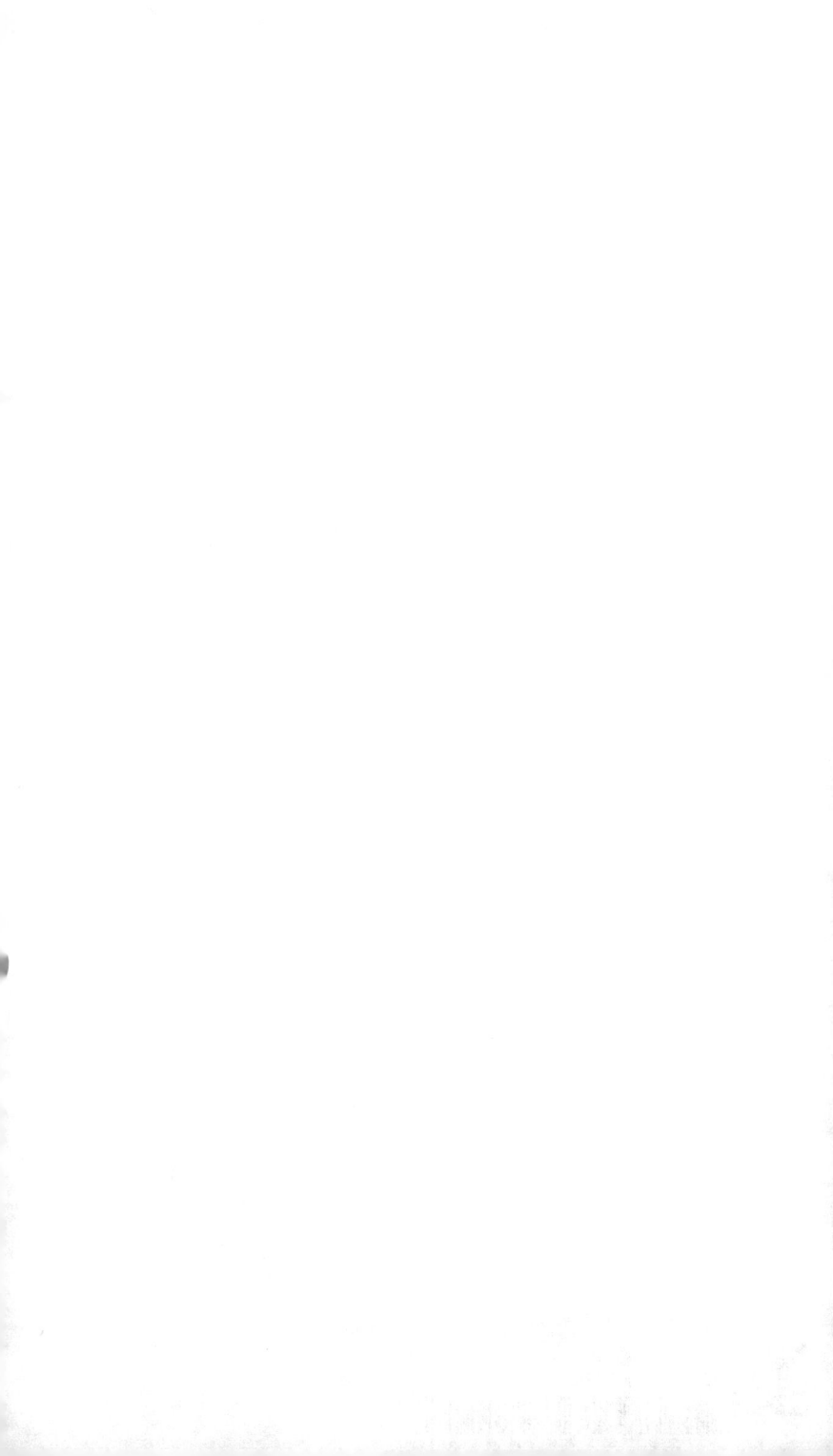

www.ingramcontent.com/pod-product-compliance
Lightning Source LLC
Chambersburg PA
CBHW070520030426
42337CB00016B/2033